Lose Weight Your Way

A quick guide to picking the diet that really suits you, and to living a healthier life

John Kott

TABLE OF CONTENTS

IN READING THIS MATERIAL

In reading this material, be very certain you never go past a word you do not fully understand. The only reason a person gives up a study or becomes confused or unable to learn and apply the information is because he or she has gone past a word that was not understood.

It may not only be the new and unusual words you have to look up. Some commonly used words can often be misdefined and so cause confusion. If you start feeling confused, or do not remember what you just read, go back and find your misunderstood words. A good old dictionary might be your best companion while reading this book.

The author is not engaged in rendering professional advice or services to the individual reader. The ideas, procedures, and suggestions contained in this book are not intended as a substitute for consulting with your physician and/or dietician. All matters regarding your health require professional supervision. The author should not be liable or responsible for any loss or damage allegedly arising from any information or suggestion in this book.

INTRODUCTION

Many of us have a habit of trying different diets from time to time, to lose weight or to have the great benefits that are associated with healthy eating. However, choosing the right diet for you is as important as following it religiously. Following the wrong diet can be as harmful as not following any at all, and in some scenarios, bad dietary habits can cause you to lose your potential and live in fear for the rest of your life. Making the right decision is very important, and it is a very rational behavior.

We must have the mentality of choosing the diet that produces the expected results in a proven way. This book will share with you five diets that actually work perfectly for losing weight and improving your overall health.

Below, you will find the benefits of a healthy diet, which you should know. Are you still worried about your weight loss regimen, or about improving your mental capacity, having amazing skin, maybe living a life without threatening diseases?

Or maybe you are looking for a reason to start with better eating habits, with drinks and meals full of nutritious elements that promote health? All of this is possible!

Well, if you want to find a unique and different diet plan that really suits you, this book is perfect. Not only are we going to talk about five regimens, but we will also discuss how you can start a better life with the help of healthy eating. This book is the "introductory package" with the information you have been searching

for a long time.
The journey to a healthy lifestyle, with the right options, is an incredible initiative, and I congratulate you on starting it. Your consideration of taking this first step is worthy of admiration! Feel proud of you taking action, while others sit on the couch not knowing what to do with themselves. I will contribute directly to your initiative, with the content of this book.
Let's start!

J.K.

CHAPTER 1

A Healthy Lifestyle

"You are what you eat."
This is one of the most fashionable phrases in our days, and it acquires more strength at every moment. Countless medical and scientific studies reinforce the claim, considering the huge health problems that arise from what we consciously or unconsciously introduce into our bodies in order to feed ourselves. From skin diseases, to chronic illnesses such as diabetes or high blood pressure, or obesity, can be caused by a poor diet.

Before going any further, let's go to basics: what does the word *diet* mean? According to the *Merriam-Webster's Dictionary*, "Diet" refers to the food and drink regularly consumed by a person, and the word comes from the Greek *"diaita"*, a manner of living and leading one's life. If you are considering switching to a healthy diet, bear in mind you will actually be shifting to a whole new way of living. It is not about making some sacrifices for some time to lose those extra pounds; it is about starting a whole new life. And it is totally worth it!

To start, let's look at the benefits of healthy eating. Some are widely known, and sometimes we seek them out more for improving our appearance than for health reasons. We will soon see that our integrity and our quality of life in general (and, therefore, that of our loved ones), depend entirely on our eating habits, and the fact of being thin or having some "little extra pounds" can be something secondary.

Benefits of a healthy diet

Weight loss

Healthy eating aids in weight loss. Healthy food is rich in nutrients (like vitamins and minerals), in contrast to "junk" food, pre-cooked meals, and other things like soft drinks, which we should eliminate from our diets. This will produce weight reduction, eventually, and keep you safe from some of the most feared chronic diseases. As the weight decreases, the chances of suffering these illnesses also diminish.

People with overweight can suffer from:

- Diabetes
- Coronary heart disease
- Complications of bone density
- Osteoarthritis (OA)
- Respiratory problems
- Various types of cancer

A healthy diet, rich in fruits and vegetables, has a much lower caloric index than that of processed foods, and the reduction of calorie consumption is essential to lose weight, because much of the energy the body does not use is stored in form of fat. One way to control what you eat, and thus lose those extra pounds, is to use a calorie counter to estimate daily consumption (there are plenty of free apps for your phone that can help you with that), and then adjust the diet plan according to the appropriate amount to achieve your goals.

A plan that completely avoids processed foods, and that limits carbohydrates, can help you stay within the proper limits and will contribute to weight reduction. Now, to manage the loss, you must also increase your fiber intake, and plant-based and vegetable-based meals contain a lot of it.

Improves your Inmune System

Your body has a natural defense system against all kinds of infections and diseases, which stops most of the bacteria and viruses that are in your environment, and that try to enter your body day after day. That barrier is the immune system. Through a series of steps, your body fights and destroys invading infectious organisms before they cause harm.

The immune process works like this: an infectious agent enters the body. Maybe it's a flu virus that enters the nose. Perhaps it is a bacterium that enters the blood when you step on a rusted nail. Your immune system is always on the alert to detect and attack the infectious agent before it causes harm. Whatever the agent, the immune system recognizes it as a foreign body. They are called antigens. And the antigens must be removed.

Our digestive health has a lot to do with the immune system. Both work closely together to keep us in good physical health. Interestingly, the immune system depends on a series of bacteria that live in our intestines, which provide essential nutrients to defend ourselves against pathogens and synthesize indigestible substances that must be expelled from the body. Likewise, it also depends on plasma, the substance in the blood responsible for transporting both nutrients to the cells and cellular waste that the body no longer needs.

Proper nutrition, with minerals and vitamins from whole, unprocessed foods, is essential for all cells to function optimally, and this includes, of course, those of the immune system.

Improves Mental Health

Mental health is very important, as much or more than the health of the body, and is necessary to live a full life. Bad moods and mood swings not only isolate you from others, they have a negative impact on our body. A healthy diet, rich in nutrients and minerals, keeps your brain in optimal conditions and balances the entire nervous system. This will keep your spirits more stable, and most important of all: in the end, you will not need to take medication to treat "mental health" problems, known for their dire side effects, regardless of the age of the person consuming them.

A healthy diet will help improve your memory and will prevent diseases such as dementia and cognitive decline when you reach advanced ages.

Improves energy

Healthy food is the perfect boost for your mood and energy. Junk food lowers your energy and you may feel drained shortly after eating. On the other hand, healthy foods raise these levels and help you stay active longer. Fruits, vegetables, seeds and grains are all part of a healthy diet, and they boost your energy so that you can be productive throughout the day.

Stress Reduction

Another wonderful benefit of a healthy diet is stress reduction. Nutritional, environmental and psychological factors play a fundamental role in managing tensions. The secret is simply a healthy diet that helps you stay calm longer, and that keeps hydrocortisone, better known as "cortisol," the stress hormone, at proper levels. As stress levels rise due to a poor diet, such as one with high amounts of refined carbohydrates and sugars, weight gain occurs because the body stores those excesses in the form of fat. This whole cycle becomes a kind of vicious circle, and breaking it might even have the same symptoms as when you quit smoking or drinking alcohol. The clearest and immediate consequences are hypertension (high blood pressure) and hyperglycemia (high blood sugar).

Improves sleep

Sleeping and having a restful sleep is very important to staying healthy. Fresh salads and other light foods are a fine source of nutrients, and do not produce a gluttony feeling.

Thus, a healthy diet reduces stomach problems and bloating. Waking up in the middle of the night from flatulence, heartburn, reflux, and other problems will be a memory of the past. This is how the right food can also improve sleep.

Prevents Dehydration

Healthy eating involves drinking a large amount of water. If you start drinking more water, you will be hydrated for longer. It has many benefits!

It improves your kidney function, keeps your body clean because it removes an enormous amount of toxic substances (such as residues of fertilizers and artificial pesticides) and helps in weight reduction, it also makes your skin healthy. However, along with consuming water, to prevent dehydration, you should eliminate sugars and refined carbohydrates (such as bread and rice).

Adults who have already reached their final growth level should drink at least 2 liters (or 1.5 gal.) of water per day. However, actual consumption will vary from person to person, depending on their weight. It is recommended to divide the person's weight in kilograms by 7, and that is the number of 250 ml. glasses the person should take. If the calculation is made in pounds and ounces, divide the number of pounds by 15, and that is the number of 8.5 oz. glasses that must be consumed.

Improves skin

Diets with healthy food are the best to obtain perfect skin. Fresh and shiny skin is very important, especially as we get older. Beauty comes from within, right? Not only in a spiritual sense, but also bodily. Therefore, if you eat healthier foods, you will surely have improved skin.

Adequate hydration and healthy meals will nourish your skin and keep it fresh. Omega 3 oil is the best to achieve this goal, and we can obtain it from some seeds, nuts, fish, and other types of food.

Reduces Cancer Possibilities

Unhealthy foods lead to obesity, and weight gain may be a step prior to the development of some forms of cancer. Although the link between one thing and the other has not been definitively established with certainty, the truth is that cancer cells reproduce more in an acidic environment, and the sugars and flours that cause weight gain also produce body acidity levels to be higher, also raising the possibility of developing this disease. A healthy diet will protect you from this malady, which can ultimately be life threatening.

Healthy natural foods like fruits, vegetables, and seeds contain antioxidants that protect cells from any damage caused by carcinogens. These are, among others:

- Beta carotene
- Lycopene
- Vitamin A
- Vitamin C
- Vitamin E

These antioxidants reduce the damage that free radicals cause to cells and lower the chances of developing cancer.

Manages diabetes

A healthy diet, full of nutrients, reduces the chances of diabetes in the person, because it helps to lose weight and controls blood sugar levels. It prevents complications from high body sugar content, and eliminates any associated symptoms such as fatigue, irritability, extreme hunger, and frequent urination. Those who already have diabetes should reduce or eliminate their intake of sugars and processed foods. So, switching to a healthy diet is actually the best option for these people.

Prevents Heart Disease

Plants and vegetables rich in vitamin E are part of a healthy diet that will help prevent heart ailments. Vitamin E reduces the possibility of heart attack, because it is vital for the strengthening of all muscles (including the heart) and the control of cholesterol in the blood. You can get it from almonds, peanuts, green vegetables, sunflower seeds and hazelnuts.

If you eliminate partially hydrogenated oils (known as trans fats, which are formed by industrially converting liquid oils to solid fats) from your diet, your cholesterol level will automatically decrease, and with it the risks of an attack.

According to scientific research, a healthy diet, combined with regular physical activity, considerably reduces the risks of heart disease, and even death, because a low cholesterol level, together with a robust heart, will ensure that there are no arterial blockages.

Lowering blood pressure plays a vital role in safeguarding anyone from heart problems. To reduce it, you must change to healthier eating habits, with low levels of carbohydrates, sugars and trans fats, and many vegetables and plants that increase the oxygen content in the blood.

Strong bones and strong teeth

Calcium, potassium and magnesium are necessary minerals to make your bones and teeth healthy, and to stay away from very painful diseases like arthritis, rheumatism, osteoporosis, and even gum disease.

Cauliflower, cabbage, low-fat dairy products, tofu, and legumes are rich in calcium and magnesium. Therefore, adding these foods to your regular diet will keep your teeth and bones strong and healthy.

Gut Health

A healthy diet promotes your stomach health and keeps it free from many intestinal diseases. The colon has a host of bacteria that live and reproduce in it naturally and are responsible for producing vital substances for your well-being. However, industrially processed foods and unsaturated fats (another name for trans fat) obstruct their production and promote inflammation in this part of the body.

For this reason, a diet enriched with vitamins, minerals and fiber, increases intestinal health and facilitates bowel movements that prevent cancer and other ills. The remains of not fully digested foods can continue its way out of the body, and as a result, the acidity levels produced by decomposing food within the large intestine are lower.

Longer life expectancy
By switching to a healthier diet, we not only prevent the onset of diseases, but also increase our life expectancy. By eliminating many of the risks of developing diseases that would put our survival at risk, we will live much longer with high quality. We will fully enjoy, with clearer senses and a better perception of everything around us.

Higher level of activity
Your energy level will be enhanced with a healthy diet, becoming more active and lowering the chances of feeling fatigued, stressed, depressed, or irritable. Your concentration to study or carry out any other activity will increase.
Eating healthy will eliminate the states mentioned above, and others, and increase your performance in any area of life.

Saves money
Finally, yet importantly, an appropriate diet is not only the best for your health; it can also be amazing for your pocket. If you prepare your food at home, your additional expenses will be surprisingly reduced overnight. A healthy diet is much cheaper than junk food or pre-processed foods, not to mention the fortune you will save by not having to buy tons of drugs to treat illnesses caused by poor nutrition throughout your entire life.

CHAPTER 2

Diets That Actually Work

People start to follow a diet to lose weight, mainly. If your intention is that, there is no problem. This is also the purpose of this book: to help you choose the best diet for you, so that you reach your ideal weight, according to your tastes, your possibilities and your lifestyle. Still, do yourself a big favor: Do not choose a diet that does not have proven positive effects. Today, you can find an overwhelming amount of information on the internet, which even offers great results in no time and with almost no effort. Take a good look at your options. Any goal worth achieving requires patience and discipline. Here are five diets that actually work perfectly for weight loss, while improving your health levels and leading you to a new life.

Option # 1: Paleo Diet

It is also known as the "Stone Age Diet". In it, the foods that have accompanied Humanity since those ancient times are consumed. Includes foods from the Paleolithic Age (roughly 3,000,000 to 12,000 years BC), which have had little or no change at all, for example: lean meats, fish, shellfish, fruits, vegetables, nuts, and seeds. The inhabitants of the Paleolithic period got their meals mainly through hunting. It also includes raw dairy foods, legumes, and grains.

The fundamental purpose when starting this diet is to return to the habits our ancestors had. Over time, technology has come to a point where the food we get from agriculture and industry has been profoundly modified, even at the genetic level. The goal of the Paleo diet is to go back to the patterns of the past to obtain benefits in our health, because modern food does not harmonize with human genes and body functions, as studies have revealed. Apparently, the body's ability to adapt to processed foods is very limited. Hence, the prevalence of diabetes, heart disease, and obesity has increased, despite the development of technologies that should have done the exact opposite. Whole foods, in contrast, help improve all body functions, mood, and overall attitude.

This diet includes a large amount of vegetables, fruits, nuts and seeds. It is one of the best to satisfy the nutritional needs of the human body. It does not make use of wheat, legumes and modified dairy products, among others. This is the main difference between the Paleo diet and other healthy regimes.

Purpose of the Paleo Diet

Here are some reasons to choose the Paleo diet:

- You can get your food more naturally
- You can lose weight
- You can prevent obesity and heart disease, as well as complications caused by the use of herbicides and pesticides.
- Meal planning is easy

What you can eat

If you plan to start the Paleo diet, we recommend that you make a daily meal plan. The following are the foods you can eat:

- Fresh fruits
- Vegetables
- Walnuts
- Seeds
- Lean meat
- Fish (especially meats rich in Omega 3 and fatty acids, such as salmon, trout and sardines)
- Olive, coconut and walnut oil
- Other oils from fruits and vegetables, such as avocado

What you should avoid

To get the most out of it, you must strictly follow the diet, and thus obtain the best results. You should avoid these foods:

- All meals with wheat
- Oatmeal
- Barley
- Pulses
- Beans
- Peanut
- Peas or peas
- Modified dairy products
- Sugar
- Salt
- Starches (like potatoes)
- Packaged and pre-processed foods

Benefits of the Paleo diet

- Raises the body's energy level.
- Helps improve sleep.
- It helps to have a clear mind and produces peace of mind.
- Does not cause inflammation or flatulence.
- There is a marked reduction in weight.
- Contributes to good muscle shape and healthy growth.
- Reduces the risk of cardiovascular disease.

- Reduces the risk of cancer and diabetes.
- Boosts the immune system.
- It has a positive effect on the way the body processes glucose.
- Improves the lipid profile and reduces insulin secretion. Lowers triglycerides (the main components of body fat).
- Reduces allergic attacks.
- It improves the respiratory system and protects the person from many respiratory illnesses.
- Contributes to control blood pressure.
- Controls appetite.

Option #2: Keto Diet

The ketogenic diet (or simply the Keto diet) is characterized by recommending the consumption of foods low in carbohydrates, but rich in fat. Those carbohydrates are replaced by high-level fats, which we find especially in red meat. Due to the reduction or elimination of carbohydrates, the body will enter a metabolic state called ketosis. In it, stored fats are broken down with the help of compounds called ketone bodies. Hence the name of the diet itself. Their main funtion is to break down fats into shorter chains, generating acetoacetate, an acid that is used as energy by the brain and the other organs of the body. In addition to helping to reduce body fat (and therefore lose weight), it also lowers glucose and insulin levels.

Types of Keto Diet

These are the types of Keto diet that you should know:

- The first type is the "Standard Ketogenic Diet". It includes low carbohydrate, high fat, and moderate protein intake.
- The second type is the "Cyclical Ketogenic Diet". This also includes high carbohydrate intake for certain periods. In a seven-day cycle, it prescribes five days of strict keto diet, and two days of high carbohydrate in-

take. The cycle repeats every week.
- The third type is the "Adapted Ketogenic Diet". Carbohydrates are added during periods of physical training.
- A high protein ketogenic diet is one in which the protein is added artificially, through supplements. It is also widely used by athletes.

The Keto diet plays an outstanding role as a method of reducing weight, while reducing the risk of fatal diseases. There is no need to keep track of calories, and it keeps you satisfied for a longer period. Weight loss can be up to 2.2 times faster than with diets that depend on daily calorie intake control. Although it may seem contradictory, it can help you lose weight faster than diets that completely avoid fats.

Keto Diet Benefits
These are the benefits of the Keto diet:

- Helps you stay more active and boosts athletic performance.
- You lose weight quickly.
- Controls glucose levels in the blood.
- It could reduce the risk of cancer.
- Improves heart health and protects brain function.
- Contributes to the decrease of acne.
- Helps reduce cramps.
- Contributes to reducing the symptoms of polycystic ovarian syndrome.
- Reduces the symptoms of Alzheimer's disease, Parkinson's and other degenerative neurological diseases.

Risks of Keto Diet
Despite all the benefits that the Keto diet can produce, this regime is not suitable for everyone, and may have the following side effects:

- Fatigue
- Keto Flu
- Constipation
- Nutritional deficiencies
- Cardiac ills (in patients with high blood pressure)
- Hypoglycemia problems
- Weight gain once the diet is stopped
- Kidney stones
- Fatty liver
- Headaches, nausea, and vomiting

Option #3: Mediterranean Diet

This diet is based on the traditional food that was consumed in the Mediterranean, especially in Italy and Greece, during the Middle Ages. It helps lose weight and has a very positive impact on heart health.

The components of the Mediterranean diet can be organized in a pyramid, depending on the recommended number of times they should be consumed during the month. At the base of the pyramid, however, there is no food, but a habit: a key part of this regimen is moderate physical activity seven days a week. In addition to that, it is recommended to consume whole grain breads, pasta, rice and other carbohydrates (also whole grains) every day, along with fruits, beans, legumes and nuts, vegetables, olive oil, cheese and yogurt. Weekly, only one serving of fish, poultry, eggs, and candy should be consumed, and lastly, red meat should be limited to one serving per month. All the above, accompanied by a minimum of six glasses of water per day.

What you can eat

The foods below are part of the Mediterranean diet:

- Vegetables and fruits
- Nuts and seeds
- Legumes and grains

- Herbs and species
- Seafood
- Dairy products in moderation
- Meats (according to the previous recommendations)
- Olive oil

What you should avoid
These foods should be avoided if you want to follow the Mediterranean diet:

- Sugars
- Meats and processed foods
- Refined grains and oils

Option #4: Intermittent Diet

The intermittent diet, also known as intermittent fasting, is very popular for losing weight almost instantly. Not only does it help achieve that goal, but it also apparently improves metabolic health and increases life expectancy. This diet is not strict as to what should be eaten but determines when it can be done and when not.

Types of fasting
Here are the basic ways you can do intermittent fasting:

- Fast for 16 hours each day.
- Fasting two days a week (the days must not be consecutive), eating less than usual.
- 24 hours fast, once or twice a week.
- Intense fast every other day.
- Fasting during the day and eating a strong meal at night.
- Avoid one mealtime a day, if this is easy for you.

Option #5: Vegan Diet

The vegan diet is one of the most popular today. In it, foods of plant origin are consumed only, such as vegetables, grains, nuts and fruits, and others that come exclusively from plants. The vegan diet does not include foods of animal origin of any kind, including dairy products and eggs. People who choose this diet do so due to several factors, mainly: health considerations, moral and ethical reasons (to avoid animal exploitation), concerns related to the environment (raising animals apparently causes high levels of CO2 and contamination of water sources), and to lose weight.

Benefits of the vegan diet

- Provides enough nutrients that the body needs on a daily basis.
- Contributes to weight loss.
- Raises energy levels throughout the day.
- Improves kidney and digestive function.
- Helps lower blood sugar level.
- Reduces the risk of cancer.
- By not consuming any type of meat, the general acidity of the body decreases.
- Contributes to the fair treatment of animals. Their rights are respected.
- Contributes to environmental preservation.

CHAPTER 3

Paleo Diet

I f you have not yet decided which weight loss regimen to follow, but want to try a unique and different plan, the Paleolithic diet is undoubtedly an excellent option for you. Many of the health problems of the 21st century find a solution with this lifestyle.

The foundations of the Paleo diet date back more than two million years. His followers argue that human anatomy, as well as its genetic design, have hardly changed since the Stone Age. Our ancestors used simpler versions of some tools, which were not suitable for planting and growing plants. For this reason, they turned to wild plants and animals to meet their food needs.

Today, some people sustain that if these ancient predecessors managed to live long enough, they may not have had the diseases of modern times, such as diabetes, heart disease, and cancer. This may be true to some extent, because along with their diet, they also engaged in intense physical activities, such as prolonged hunting periods, and their meals were mainly uncooked lean meats and plants. Currently, we know that physical exercise is one of the fundamental habits to live healthier, in an adequate weight range. Due to all the above, life expectancy of our ancestors might have been very high.

The Paleo diet began to become well known around 2014, at-

tracting its followers and motivating them to eat healthy. They quickly became interested in learning about the power sources of Stone Age women and men.
Let's look at the basic information about the Paleo diet:

What is the Paleo diet?

For sure, you are wondering what exactly the Paleo diet is. The design of this regime bears resemblance to what we believe was the diet of our ancestors of the Paleolithic era. Their diet was that of hunters and gatherers. Despite this, one cannot clearly imagine what these first humans could have eaten across the planet. The researchers argue that most of their foods were whole foods.
Hunters had physically very active lives, and their diets had the mentioned basis. Apparently, it kept them safe from chronic diseases, and of course from obesity. Many studies indicate that this diet achieves a very significant effect in weight loss.

How It Works

The "Caveman Diet," as it is also known, includes fish, seeds, lean meats, vegetables, fruits, and nuts. His followers point out that you must choose foods that do not raise the glycemic index (this is the ability a food has to raise the blood sugar level, such as refined flours). The most recommended are fruits and vegetables.
The debate about what foods were truly available in that era continues. A point on which there is still no agreement is that of the possible variations that existed in the diets, depending on the area where the Paleolithic women and men lived. It could not have been the same diet for the inhabitants of the Arctic regions, as for those of the Tropics. Additionally, there are notable differences between the fruits and vegetables of those times, and those of modern times. Experts still do not agree on whether they should rather be excluded from the diet. For all the above, there is no single version of the Paleo diet. An example of this is white potatoes. This food was already available during the Paleolithic

period; however, they are currently avoided, due to their elevated glycemic index.

In general, the Paleo diet has a high proportion of protein, moderation with respect to fats (those consumed are mainly those naturally contained in food), and moderation with carbohydrates. Try a high fiber intake, and a low intake of sugars and sodium. You must bear in mind that the followers of this diet obtain mono-unsaturated and polyunsaturated fats, such as docosahexaenoic acid and eicosapentaenoic acid, derived from Omega-3 (DHA and EPA), from seeds, marine fish, nuts, avocado and olive oil. They avoid eating processed foods, due to the emphasis given to fresh foods, in the most natural condition possible. Some people make use of frozen fruits and vegetables, since many of the nutrients are still present without deterioration despite the freezing process.

The Paleo diet highlights the preference for grazing beef over industrial meat produced by conventional means, because it contains higher levels of Omega-3, in the form of alpha linolenic acid (ALA). Additionally, conventional beef comes from grain-fed animals, most likely with genetically modified corn. Small amounts of DHA and EPA, as well as ALA, also derived from Omega-3, are present in the Paleo diet. Still, levels of Omega oils are considerably higher in wild (non-farmed) marine fish than in grazing beef. For example, a three-ounce piece of cooked salmon has between 1000 and 2000 mg of EPA / DHA, while a similar serving of grazing beef contains only 20 to 200 mg of ALA.

Some pointers

- Proponents of the Paleo diet prefer to consume fresh lean meat, seeds, fruits, fish (wild, not farmed), nuts, shellfish, coconut and olive oils, and small amounts of honey as a sweetener.
- If you follow this diet, you should remember that it is preferable to avoid sugars, cereals, modified dairy products, legumes such as lentils, beans and peanuts, coffee, and refined oils such as canola, and potatoes. Processed

foods, even if they are labelled "healthy", are also not recommended.

- There is no set daily calorie count or set portion sizes. If you are disciplined enough, you can even eat a few "cheat" meals during the week, particularly at the start of the regimen, so sticking to the rules is a little easier. You can afford a little wine or dark chocolate. Red wine and chocolate with a cocoa content of 70% or more have a high amount of nutrients and antioxidants. They are nutritious and beneficial.

Recommended foods

There is no one way to follow the Paleo diet for everyone. The inhabitants of the Paleolithic managed to prosper with different combinations, depending on what was available in the various areas and periods. Some consumed few carbohydrates and large amounts of animal-derived foods, and others turned to plants high in carbohydrates, such as tubers. This information is primarily a guide for those who follow the diet, not something set in stone. You could even include brown rice and grazing cow's butter if you want. You can make changes and adapt it according to your needs, tastes and preferences.

You can consume healthy fats (as they are naturally found, unprocessed), nuts, eggs, fruits and vegetables, fish, herbs, meats, condiments, and seeds. Be sure to include pork, beef, turkey, chicken, and lamb, among others, and wild (non-farmed) fish and shellfish like trout, salmon, shrimp, and mackerel. Remember to look for animal products obtained in the most natural way possible; industrial farm production generally relies on genetically modified grain-based animal feed. Also include vegetables such as tomatoes, broccoli, carrots, onions, peppers, and lettuce.

Try to avoid processed foods, trans fats, vegetable oils, legumes, margarine, carbonated beverages, and artificial sweeteners (such as acesulfame K, aspartame, saccharin, and sucralose), as well as modified dairy products. Of course, all foods that contain corn syrup and sugar, such as candy, ice cream, any type of pastry, and commercial fruit juices, should not be consumed.

Even some grains and foods based on them, such as barley, wheat, rye, spelled, breads, and pasta, are not allowed, as are low-fat processed dairy products. However, in some Paleo trends, whole dairy like butter and cheese are accepted. As already mentioned, you should avoid vegetable oils such as grapeseed, corn, cottonseed, soy or sunflower seed oil, and the trans fats present in prepared meals. Margarine, both in its hydrogenated and partially hydrogenated version, is also not recommended.

The golden rule is simple, for this and for all other diets: do not eat factory-produced food. It cannot be easier than that. Be sure to read all the ingredients on the list in industrial foods, even if the packaging claims to be "healthy food."

CHAPTER 4

Keto Diet

The "Keto diet" is known for being low in carbohydrates and rich in fats, with a moderate consumption of protein. In the "Keto" or ketogenic diet, the calories necessary for functioning are completed using high-fat foods, such as some red meats. It keeps you hydrated, more satisfied, improves your mood and your level of activity, making you have more energy throughout the day.

According to traditional scientific research, the primary source of energy for the human body comes from carbohydrates, molecules composed mainly of carbon, hydrogen and oxygen, which may have other elements, such as sulfur, phosphorous and nitrogen. However, when a body does not receive these carbohydrates, it is able to transform the stored fat (in your abdomen, your hips, your limbs, etc.) into energy. Compounds called ketone bodies are generated (hence the name ketogenic), which break down fat into shorter chains, in the liver, producing acetoacetic acid, fuel for the brain and the rest of the body. Thus, it is clear that the body can obtain its energy not only from carbohydrates, but also from fats. For this reason, a natural metabolic process, such as ketosis, is used in some of the most effective diets for weight reduction, eliminating additional body fat.

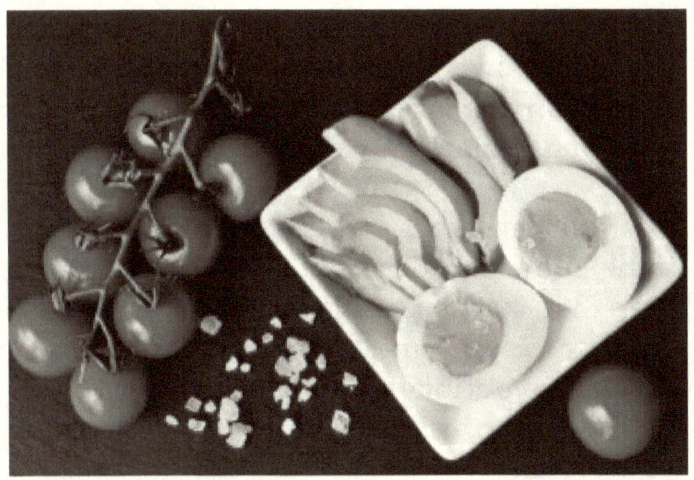

Some studies also state that blood sugar levels in patients with type I and II diabetes are better controlled through a ketogenic diet. By reducing the consumption of carbohydrates, which thanks to metabolism would be converted to sugars, the need for insulin in the body also decreases and glucose levels stabilize, without requiring additional medication. There are studies that point out the benefits of the Keto diet for patients with conditions such as Alzheimer's disease and epilepsy that do not respond favorably to regular pharmacology. We cannot forget that, in the beginning, the ketogenic diet was born as an effort to treat neurological diseases, such as epilepsy, because of the way it helps to energize the brain. Despite the great results it has had, the scientific studies are not entirely conclusive regarding the real scope of the Keto diet.

How to switch to a Keto diet

Here are some tips to keep in mind before starting a Keto diet:

- First, you must gain a thorough understanding of which foods are carbohydrates, which are fats, and which are proteins, and how they affect your body. There is a wealth of literature and audiovisual resources on these topics, both in traditional and online media. To avoid problems, always turn to authorized and professional sources on the subject.

- You must know which fats are good, and the role they play.
- If your main diet consists of prepared meals, or even "junk" food, and you want to start a healthy diet, like the Keto diet, start by eating salads. Increase plant-derived foods and fat-rich meat intake gradually, until you completely discontinue previous habits.
- Reduces the intake of sugars. Eat sweet fruits to calm your cravings.
- The first week is always the hardest, no matter when you start. However, you must be consistent and ignore symptoms such as fatigue, or headaches that happen at first. Remember that you are breaking a vicious circle. Sugars and flours have the same effects on the body and mind as a vice, such as smoking or alcoholism. You are not going to die, and those symptoms will disappear over time.
- The most important tip is to select the right foods that perfectly meet your energy needs. Add new foods to your routine gradually, until you have completely changed to the new diet.

Many of the people who are obese and want to lose weight, choose this diet. Additionally, the Keto diet is also beneficial in preventing high-risk heart conditions. Reduces the likelihood of seizures, brain and neural diseases, skin and intestinal problems, and others. As mentioned above, you should speak to your doctor and consult before starting the ketogenic diet, or any other diet.

Types of Keto Diet

These are the main types of Keto diets:

- The first is the "Standard Ketogenic Diet" (SKD). It comprises few carbohydrates, moderate protein and high fat foods. In total, the fat percentage should be 75%, while carbohydrates should not exceed 5%. The rest should be protein.
- The second type is the "Cyclic Ketogenic Diet". Includes high carbohydrate refills. This means that a strict Keto diet must be followed for five days a week, and a high carbohydrate diet for two days, and the cycle is repeated every week.
- The next type is the "Adapted Ketogenic Diet". This is ideal for athletes who do specialized physical activity as part of their daily routine. Carbohydrate consumption is allowed only 30 minutes before, during, and 30 minutes after the training session.
- The last type is the "High Protein Ketogenic Diet". As its name implies, protein consumption is here higher than usual. In SKD, intake should be around 20%. With a Keto diet high in protein, the percentage rises to at least 30%, which must be obtained from animal sources or from seeds.

The "Standard Ketogenic Diet" is the most recommended one by researchers and specialists.

What you can eat

This is a list of the foods that can be consumed as part of the Keto diet:

- Beef, pork and poultry (main foods)
- Fish and seafood
- Low carbohydrate vegetables
- Low carb cheeses
- Avocado
- Coconut and olive oil

- Eggs
- Low carb yogurt (like Greek yogurt) or cottage cheese
- Nuts and seeds
- Berry fruits (strawberries, raspberries, blackberries, etc.)
- Butter
- Low carb pasta (including shirataki noodles)
- Olives
- Coffee and tea without sugar
- Whipped cream
- Dark chocolate and cocoa powder.

As you can see, you can eat a wide variety of tasty and nutritious foods in a ketogenic regime. Try to vary between vegetables and meats for extended seasons, so you can get all the necessary nutrients.

What you should avoid
These foods should be avoided when following a Keto diet:

- Beans and peas
- Peanuts
- Low fat dairy derivatives
- Rice and pasta
- Artificial sweeteners
- Foods with added sugars
- Processed fruit juices
- Soft and flavored drinks
- Sandwiches
- Sweet fruits
- Starches (such as tubers)
- Trans fats
- Alcoholic drinks

Keto Snacks
If you need a snack between two heavy mealtimes, the Keto diet has several options:

- Chunks of meat or fish
- Nuts or seeds
- Cheese with olives
- Cooked eggs
- Dark chocolate (90% cocoa)
- Low carbohydrate protein shakes
- Whole yogurt
- Strawberries
- Whipped cream

Supplements

If necessary, the Keto diet also considers some food supplements that can be added. This is a small list:

- Medium Chain Triglyceride Oil (MTC)
- Minerals
- Caffeine
- Creatine
- Whey protein, from animal sources
- Exogenous ketones

Benefits

In addition to aiding in weight loss, and kick-starting your metabolism for energy, there are other benefits of following a Keto diet. Here we summarize some:

- Strengthens skin health and reduces acne.
- Reduces the chances of cancer.
- Improves heart health and brain function.
- Reduces the possibility of involuntary muscle contractions, or cramps.
- Helps reduce polycystic ovarian symptoms.
- Boosts mental health.

Possible Side Effects

As we mentioned earlier, changing your eating habits can have adverse effects on the body, which is why it is always better to be under the supervision of a nutrition professional who can quickly assess anything that happens. Despite its enormous benefits, the Keto diet can subject the body to stress, and some of these situations can arise:

- Kidney stones
- Increased protein level in the blood
- Deficiency of minerals or vitamins
- Constipation
- Fatigue
- Headaches and vomiting
- Decreased aerobic capacity of the body
- Development of fatty liver

In conclusion, we have discussed the Keto diet extensively, and now we know a little better about its effects on our bodies and our lifestyle. It has enormous benefits, such as its contribution to reducing the chances of cancer, diabetes and other diseases. We also know that it can have some adverse effects, which a professional in the field could quickly detect and correct. Switching to a Keto diet will not only help you control your weight, eliminating all that extra fat; it may be the start of a new life.

CHAPTER 5

Mediterranean Diet

The Mediterranean diet includes traditional foods from the Mediterranean countries, mainly Greece and Italy, as it is believed they were consumed in the Middle Ages (approx. 475 to 1450 AD), in the times of the Roman Empire. It became popular again in the 1960s, when researchers found that people in that area generally had considerably better health than the people that lived in the United States.

With this diet, the risks of contracting many of the modern diseases caused by day-to-day routines are very low. Many studies also revealed that the Mediterranean diet produces weight loss. It also proves to be beneficial in preventing premature deaths, type II diabetes, and fulminant heart attacks.

You cannot determine a unique and specific way to follow this diet, because there are many countries, with particular customs, around the Mediterranean Sea. People living in these countries consume different foods, nevertheless around a similar eating philosophy.

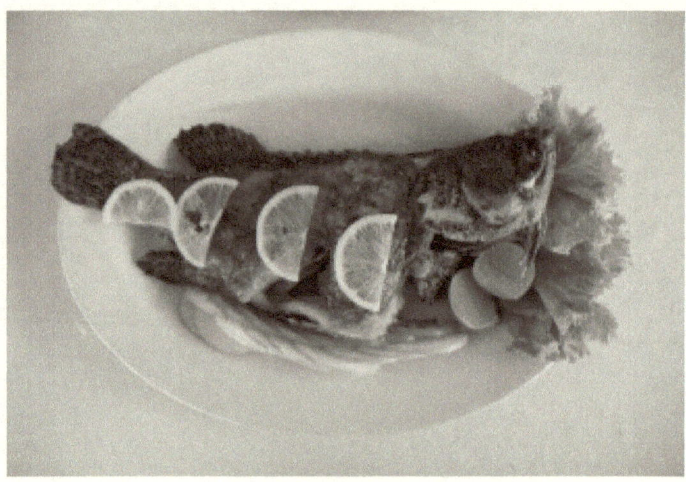

The Basics

The Mediterranean diet comprises many food groups. You can eat vegetables, nuts, fruits, potatoes and legumes, portions of bread, whole grains, seeds, herbs, seafood, condiments, extra virgin olive oil and fish. You can also eat poultry, yogurt, eggs, and cheese in moderation. You can eat red meat very occasionally. Make sure you do not drink beverages with added sugars. Avoid them entirely, as well as refined grains and oils, and processed foods, including sausages and the like. Keep in mind that regular sugar, carbonated drinks, ice creams and sweets are also not recommended. Refined flours, used to make all kinds of breads and pastries, and pasta made from refined wheat, are part of the foods to avoid. Products labeled "diet" or "low fat" should also not be consumed. Any product that comes from an industrial process will be harmful to health. Always read labels for unhealthy artificial ingredients.

What you can eat

There has been a wide debate to decide which foods belong to the Mediterranean diet. It does not have a specific plan, and this makes it a controversial topic. The reason, as explained above, is that the countries around the Mediterranean Sea are many, and each region has its own ancient traditions.

Studies suggest that various of those regional diets are rich in plant-based options, which are very healthy. Animal sources are rather limited. Still, eating seafood and fish twice a week is recommended.

An important point, if we look at the Mediterranean lifestyle, is that they do some physical exercise on a regular basis and enjoy sharing life and mealtimes with family and friends. Actually, they take the time to sit down and eat calmly, in contrast to our hectic pace of life.

If you follow the Mediterranean diet, be sure to include vegetables like cucumber, broccoli, tomatoes, cauliflower, kale (a variety of cabbage that has deep green leaves, seems to be a mix between lettuce, Swiss chard and broccoli), Brussels sprouts, carrots, onions and spinach.

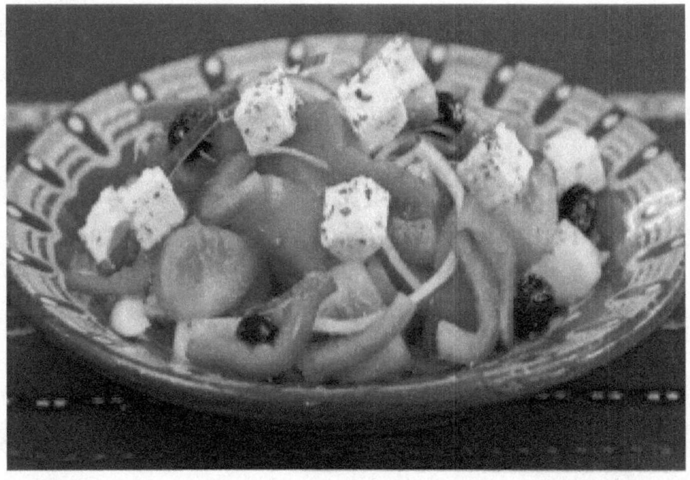

You can enjoy apples, peaches, bananas, melons, figs, oranges, grapes, strawberries, and pears. You can complement them with nuts and seeds such as pumpkin, almonds, sunflower and cashew seeds, and hazelnuts. Legumes, such as peas, chickpeas, beans and lentils, are also recommended in the Mediterranean diet.

In this diet, tubers such as turnips, potatoes and sweet potatoes are accepted. Recommended whole grains are whole oats, rye, buckwheat, brown rice, corn, and barley. Of course, whole wheat pasta and bread are also part of the diet. Chicken, turkey, and duck meat is acceptable, as are the eggs of those animals, along with quail.

Fish and shellfish are also part of this eating style. Mussels, salmon, tuna, sardines and mackerel, trout, oysters, crabs, shrimp and clams, among others, are characteristic of the Mediterranean cuisine, especially if they are seasoned with herbs and spices (pepper, garlic, basil, cinnamon, mint, nutmeg, sage and rosemary, etc.). Finally, you can add dairy products, such as Greek or plain yogurt, and a variety of cheeses. A little extra virgin olive oil, or avocado (in oil or whole), and a few olives, will make your meals even healthier and tastier.

What should you drink?

Water is the main drink in the Mediterranean diet, and you should consume a minimum of six 250 ml (8.5 oz) glasses a day. You can drink red wine in moderation, without exceeding a glass a day.

Of course, remember this is not mandatory and can change. You should definitely avoid wine, or any alcoholic beverage if you cannot control alcohol consumption. Coffee or tea is always an option. The main thing is that you do not drink beverages that have added sugars. Use natural fruit juices instead.

If you are on the Mediterranean diet, you should not have more than three meals a day. However, there are some snack options to hold between one time and another:

- A handful of any type of walnuts
- Apple bits with almond butter
- A portion of fruit, or carrot
- Greek yogurt
- Some grapes or berries

This diet is very appropriate if you go out to eat at a restaurant. You can order any seafood or fish as your main course, and you only must ask them to prepare it with extra virgin olive oil, not with butter, much less with margarine or refined oils. To accompany, ask for whole wheat bread with a little olive oil.

Final remarks

If you decide to follow the Mediterranean diet, buy only in stores that offer whole foods. Buy as few processed foods as possible. Sure, organic groceries are the best option, but sometimes they are not as accessible. They may have high prices. However, it is worth investing in quality food.

Get all low-quality, processed foods out of your kitchen and out of the refrigerator. If you run out of harmful options, you will *finally* eat healthy food. Do not be considerate of yourself.

The Mediterranean diet does not have a unique design, and yet it is rich in nutrients that come from plants, seafood and fish. It does not make extensive use of red meat. It is very attractive and healthy, and surely you will not be disappointed.

CHAPTER 6

Intermittent Fasting

In the contemporary world, Intermittent Fasting (IF) is among the most popular trends for staying fit. It gained popularity almost instantly. Its effectiveness in losing weight and improving health in general have drawn a lot of attention, not to mention the way it can simplify our lives.

Many studies support the fact that IF has very powerful effects on the brain and body. It could even increase our life expectancy.

More than a diet itself, IF is a different eating pattern. It comprises eating cycles combined with fasting cycles. What the person eats is not important in this diet, although of course, it is suggested the same considerations be taken as with the previous diets: no processed food, no sugars and refined flours, no trans-fat, etc. The IF concentrates on the moments the person should eat. The standard IF method contemplates a daily fast of 16 hours. If the person can tolerate even a 24-hour fast without a break, it is best to do it only twice a week.

During millions of years of evolution, fasting was a common practice of Humanity until relatively recently. Hunters and gatherers of Prehistory had no means for storing their food, and their availability varied widely throughout the year. Sometimes they could not eat anything at all, simply because there was nothing to eat. What could these men and women do? They had no choice but to fast, and this enabled them to survive without food for longer periods. Fasting is natural for humans, instead of having several meals throughout the day.

Finally, many religions, such as Christianity, Buddhism, Judaism and Islam, have fasting within their precepts, as a way of purifying the body and spirit, in order to have a better relationship with the Supreme Being.

Intermittent Fasting Methods

There are many ways to follow IF. They consist of dividing the days and weeks into periods of feeding and fasting, alternately. During the latter, the idea is not to eat at all, or to eat very little. The most popular methods are:

The 16/8 method: It is also known as the *Leangains* method, created by personal trainer and nutritionist Martin Berkhan. In it, the person does not eat daily breakfast and restricts all meals for the day to an eight-hour period, followed by 16 hours of fasting. The body, by depleting all the glucose ingested, initiates ketosis to obtain the necessary energy, a process that we already explained extensively in Chapter 4 of this book. It is an excellent method of gaining muscle mass (hence the name *lean gains*).

Eat - Stop - Eat: Here you must fast for 24 hours straight, once or twice a week. For example: you do not eat from dinner one day until dinner the next day. If you decide to fast in this way twice a week, it is recommended not to fast on consecutive days.

The 5:2 diet: This pattern allows the consumption of only 500-600 calories on two days of the week. They do not need to be consecutive. You can eat as usual in the remaining five days.

It is certain that with the reduced consumption of calories your weight will also decrease. These eating patterns will help you in that adventure, as long as you do not exceed your intake (of carbs and sugars especially) during the periods that you can eat. The 16/8 method is the most popular, and the simplest, and we recommend that you start with that one if you decide to do IF.

How It Affects Your Cells

Fasting is not just a possibility to improve life in general. As we will see later, it may be a necessary practice.

During fasting, your body goes through a series of cellular and molecular changes. Hormone levels are adjusted to make use of stored fats and increase their availability. Cells start a repair process, and even some genetic traits change. The human growth hormone (HGH), responsible for growth and metabolism, because it allows protein uptake and muscle strengthening, increases its production up to five times, in relation to the periods in which you eat regularly. The loss of weight and the growth of muscle mass then becomes evident, in addition to which insulin levels are reduced. A high insulin content in the blood can cause minor problems, such as anxiety and hunger, but can eventually lead to more severe problems, such as pancreatic cancer or severe seizures.

Cell repair begins during fasting periods. This process is called autophagy. It is a regulated cell mechanism that allows for the orderly degradation and recycling of cellular components that are no longer needed or functional. This mechanism then offers protection from many diseases, and an effect of greater longevity in cells and genes.

All of these are the benefits of IF.

A Weight Loss Tool

Most people try IF to lose weight. Calorie intake is significantly reduced due to less food being eaten, and this produces hormonal changes that support weight loss.

In addition to helping to trigger ketosis, it increases the release of norepinephrine. This hormone slightly increases heart rate and pressure, and therefore blood flow throughout the body. The body requires more energy, which is then synthesized from stored fats. That is why it is also considered a "fat-burning" hormone. Even the speed of metabolism improves.

Now, a reminder: fasting will contribute to weight loss only if you consume fewer calories from carbohydrates. If you eat more than usual during the allowed periods, you will not lose the accumulated fat and you will continue to have the same appearance, along with the same health problems. You will not reach the proposed goals.

IF has many benefits beyond weight loss, as we have already seen. Achieving a healthy body and mind is among the first. It also increases your life expectancy, reduces insulin resistance drastically, and controls the production of that hormone, a situation that will protect you from type II diabetes.

The inflammation caused by some chronic diseases decreases or disappears. Low-density lipoproteins (LDLs), known as "bad cholesterol," and some indicators of inflammation, such as the sedimentation rate of erythrocytes (red blood cells), C-reactive protein and plasma viscosity, blood sugar level and triglycerides, also reach the appropriate levels.

Metabolism reaches its optimal functioning, thus preventing the appearance of diseases such as cancer. The brain-derived neurotrophic factor protein (BDNF), which causes the development and growth of the nervous system, increases its production, thus preventing the appearance of diseases such as Alzheimer's and others of a mental nature. The anti-aging effects are also obvious.

CHAPTER 7

Vegan Diet

The Vegan diet is very popular today. People are starting more and more with this regimen due to health, environmental and ethical considerations. If you follow it correctly, it will bring you many benefits.

First of all, you are going to see with satisfaction how your waist and belly get smaller. However, being entirely plant-based, you may develop a deficiency of some nutrients. It will not be anything serious if you handle it on time.

This section provides an adequate guide to start a vegan diet. It covers the most important details so you can follow it without problems.

What is the Vegan Diet?

Maybe you have heard someone talking about "veganism". It is simply a lifestyle in which the person excludes all consumer objects of animal origin, without exception. It doesn't matter if they are clothing, food or if they have another purpose.

For this reason, and unlike some vegetarian trends, vegans do not consume dairy products, eggs, or any type of meat.

There are many reasons that lead people to follow vegan philosophy, ranging from environmental considerations to ethical concerns. However, you should keep in mind that these reasons also come from a very strong desire to achieve a full life, improving overall health.

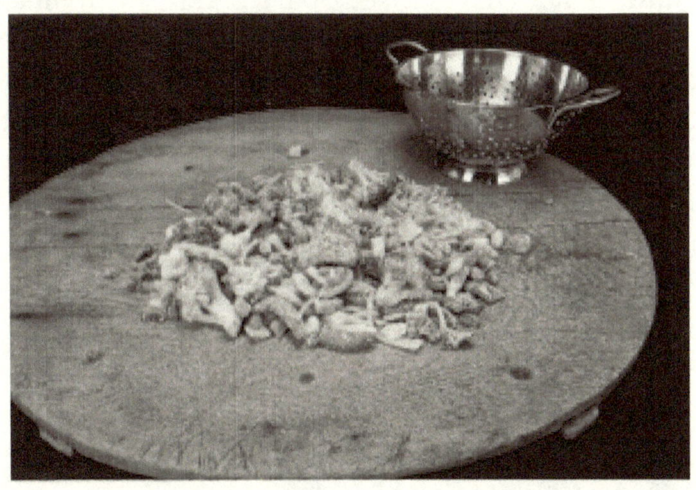

Different Types of Vegan Diets

Vegan food trends have a great variety. We present you some of the most common diets:

Whole - Food Vegan Diet: it includes a wide variety of integral products, such as seeds, legumes, nuts, fruits, vegetables and whole grains, consumed without cooking.

80/10/10: This diet includes plants, seeds, nuts, raw fruits and vegetables. Cooking temperature must be below 48 ° C (118 ° F). Its name is due to the recommendation to eat up to 80% of calories from carbohydrates, 10% from protein and the remaining 10% from fat. Limit the amount of foods such as avocados and nuts, due to its high fat content. To replace them, fleshy green plants and fruits, such as bananas, are recommended

The Starch Solution: this option is similar to the previous one. It is a diet of high carbohydrates and little vegetable fat. Emphasis is placed on cooked starches, such as potatoes, rice, and corn (the latter whole grains, of course). Fruits are not consumed.

Raw Till 4: this is another low-fat option. It is a combination of the other vegan possibilities. Raw foods are eaten every day until 4:00 pm, and dinner consists of cooked plants.

Vegan "Junk" Diet: this is a very particular option and accepts several exceptions. Unlike the others, it does not make use of whole foods exclusively, and you can eat cheeses. It also allows vegan desserts, potato chips, imitation meats, and other processed vegan foods. Strictly speaking, it cannot be said to be a true vegan diet, but there are still experts who include it in this group.

You can see the small differences between the various types, but researchers consider them as part of a single trend.

Vegans generally have a low body mass index, compared to people who are not. This index is a relationship between the weight and height of a person. The more weight a person has, the higher the BMI, which should ideally be between 18.5 and 25. The possibility of having the ideal weight is the main reason that many people choose this lifestyle. However, there are other factors: Vegans do regular physical activities and prefer alternative means of transportation, such as walking or riding a bicycle. Their decisions are based on an intention to improve overall health, and to protect the environment in a broader sense. Researchers have observed that those who start a vegan diet lose weight faster, even when they decide to eat as much as they want until they are really satisfied. High fiber intake allows the feeling of fullness to last longer.

Blood sugar reaches adequate levels, which is why the insulin the body produces can do its job better, let alone heart health. Your heart will stay healthy for much longer.

CONCLUSION

A healthy diet is absolutely the best option! Such a lifestyle is not only wonderful for your well-being, it will also save you a lot of money, and the benefits will be obvious to yourself, your coworkers, and the people around you and who you care about. When we prepare our own meals, and use natural, unprocessed ingredients, such as fruits, meats, and vegetables, we actually take control of our nutrition, thereby reducing the addition of harmful substances, from ordinary sugar to chemicals that poison us.

A healthy diet prevents all kinds of chronic, digestive, mental and degenerative diseases, whose treatments can cost thousands of dollars each month.

Therefore, having a healthy lifestyle can be the best for your economy as well, although at first it seems more expensive.

Finally, I present you a short summary of each of the diets discussed in this book:

Paleolithic Diet: does not admit the use of processed foods, rather advises the use of foods of plant and animal origin. It is possible to consume brown rice, hopefully gluten-free, and butter from pasture-raised animals. It has several versions, so you can choose the one that best suits your needs.

Ketogenic Diet: it has various beneficial effects on your lifestyle, especially for your general health. In addition to burning stored fats quickly, it reduces the risk of cancer, diabetes, and other ills.

It is based on very little or no carbohydrate consumption, and high amounts of fatty foods.

Mediterranean Diet: does not follow a certain pattern or design. It is based on plants and fish/shellfish, poultry, and a very small portion of red meat. Fruits and seeds, along with whole grains, are also part of this diet. Moderate physical activity is an integral part of this regimen.

Intermittent Fasting: it is surprising for several reasons. It does not determine what to eat, but the times of the day or week when you can do it. The management of insulin in the body improves considerably and reaches optimal levels. The same goes for cholesterol, triglycerides, and blood sugar. This leads to lower chances of developing diabetes, especially type II, reduces inflammation of the entire body, as well as the appearance of chronic diseases. It favors the growth of nerve cells, which protects against Alzheimer's and other diseases associated with old age. The anti-aging effects will also be obvious.

Vegan Diet: one of the most popular today; only strictly plant-based products are consumed, be they food or commonly used goods. Ideal for losing accumulated fat and cleaning the body, it also contributes to guaranteeing the proper treatment of animals and the conservation of the environment.

Regardless of which diet you decide to follow from now on, there are some common traits among all healthy options: avoid sugars, prepared pre-processed foods, and refined carbohydrates in all their forms. Any food that comes from the mainstream food industry has been profoundly modified, to the point that it is impossible to know what is still natural and what is artificial, genetically modified. Our bodies have undergone millions of years of evolution, and in less than a century our eating patterns have changed dramatically, most of the time towards the worst. It is no surprise then that we are having so many health problems from eating, of which being overweight is just one. Paradoxically, we could even say that being overweight is actually a reflection of how poorly we eat.

Now you know simple, very basic, but very valuable information. Deepen your knowledge about any of the diets we have covered, or other options you find. The Internet is an inexhaustible source of data, and it is vital that you adopt only the best for your daily life. Go to reliable sources, and consult with a nutrition expert whenever you can, who will accompany you throughout the process. Regardless of the diet you follow, pay close attention to the signals your body communicates to you. Your body will clearly indicate which ingredients in the diet are "friendly" and which are "aggressors" that cause undesirable effects. Unfortunately, there will be many of your favorite foods that will have this "aggressive" nature. In those cases, you should use the best of your discipline to consciously avoid them. Your health is more important than any passing craving.

Take responsibility for the health of your body and mind right now, and that of your family and loved ones around you. Start by changing some of the things you need every day, which are your source of energy, without which you cannot do nothing else: your food.

9 7 9 8 6 3 5 3 4 3 7 4 6